FLESH AND BLOOD: THE JOURNEY OF A SINGLE DAD

ANTHONNIE EASON

PUBLISHED BY BAM! PUBLISHING

Flesh and Blood: The Journey of a Single Dad

First Edition

Print edition ISBN: 9781631114694

Printed in the United States of America

TABLE OF CONTENTS

This book is dedicated to my Pride and Joy, my FLESH AND BLOOD, DJ and Adriana (Adri). They are smart, driven, confident, and in my daughter's words, "ready to shine."

To the men who are fighting for custody of their kids and/or seeking more time with their children, I applaud you beyond any words I could ever write. Continue to fight for your kids, and seek out those support systems that can assist you!

Contributors for this book are:
DENNIS JACKSON SR
LOUISE TURNER
ROBYN CALIFORNIA
J. KEVIN MCINTYRE

ACKNOWLEDGEMENTS

I'd be remiss if I didn't thank a number of people that helped me with this project. It was important to me that I do more than just relay a bunch of my experiences. I wanted to provide the perspective of others that I knew a reader could identify with. You either planted a seed, answered my calls, or pushed this book over the finish line. Thank you!

Peter "Spyder" Parker^
Maurice Reynolds^
Andrae Ballard^
J Kevin*
Monica Yoas^
Robyn*
Alicia Jett^
Louise M. Turner*
Christina Pettus^
Mark Cohen^
Dennis Jackson Sr*
Jason Mathews^
Kaoi Mathews^
Isha Haley^
Brand Kroeger^

^ Advisors
* Contributors – See Chapter 7

Acknowledgements

The names on this list are people who helped me in some shape or form, get through a tough divorce for the sake of my kids. Others on this list didn't say a word, but over the years they simply displayed the difference between fathering a child and being a daddy regardless of who was watching. Thanks for setting the example!

Hubert C. Eason Sr
Albert Andrews
Hubert C. Eason Jr
John Eason
Len Goff
Labon Eason
W. Montague Winfield
Al Ray Andrews
Robert Eason
Johnny Robertson Sr
Marshall Johnson
Sylvester Winston
Dennis Nash Sr
Vincent Williams
Maurice Reynolds
Calvin "Buster" Redd
Kenneth Harris
Johnny Hall
DJ Andrews
Dennis Nash, Jr
Johnny Roberson Jr
Kelvin Rhodes Sr
Terry McCauley Sr
Terry McCauley Jr
Dwayne Redd Jr
Robert Gerald
Robert Ray
Alphonso Lawrence

Rodger Winston
Damon Gillians
Andrae Ballard
Tommy "Hitman" Spikes
Richard Wilson
Chuck Harris
Dennis Jackson Sr
Larry "Thrill" Hill
Damon King
Al "Byrd" Williams
Alex Robinson
Pierre Perry
Welbon Monroe
Thomas Shelton
Calvin Neal
James McKay III
Chris Amos
Louis Blakey
Dave Heard
Sonny Freemon
Rynele Mardis
Emm Jay
Peter "Spyder" Parker
Efrem Gause
Jared Harty
Damien Cunningham
Claiborne Young
Edrick McDonald
Christopher Washington
David Lyles
Jason Matthews
Mark Cohen
Tyrone Birchfield
Daryl Strong
J Kev McEntyre
Conway Ekpo
Arthur Griffin
Kevin Collins
Jasey Briley
Kevin Wilkinson

Xavier Brunson
Michael Garrett
Lava the Barber
Alfie Roberts
Christopher Duke
Sean Stigler
Keith Saddler
Matt Green
Earl "Esko" Smith
Mo "Twin Boys" Robinson
Koai Mathews
Hugh Campbell
Bernard Fox
"Stormin" Norman Simon
James Porter
Emajii Graves
Conrad Farmer
Anthony Pennington
Kelly Robinson
Bryan Shaw
Chad Bass
K. Leonardus Smith Sr

FOREWORD

About two years ago (Jan 2016), I was inspired by a number of individuals who expressed themselves vocally on things they were passionate about and ultimately published books to spread their views to the masses. Everyday life has gotten in the way of completing this book, but I've had plenty of motivation in recent months to finish this project. Up front, I'd like to caveat that it is not my intent to smear or bash any single mother who's breaking her back to raise one or multiple children on her own. In my early childhood, my Dad worked 6-7 days per week, 12 hours each shift to provide for our family. It was my mother, who cooked and fed my sister and me. It was my mother that showed us how to clean, do laundry, and treat people with respect. Moreover, I applaud the efforts of those mothers whose relationship/marriage didn't work out with the father but understand how vital it is to respectfully co-parent in a non-dramatic fashion. <u>Those women get the fact that KIDS NEED THEIR DADS – and I wish there were more of them.</u>

This book IS intended to reach anyone who thinks men are not as capable as women to raise children, or those women who keep children from their dads due to relationship differences such as divorce and other related reasons. As doubts and assumptions that men are not capable or willing to parent arise, I ask that my readers stop and truly assess what they are saying. If there are no such examples in their circles of life, use me and those in this book as a reference for what real dads are and what real dads do with and for their kids each and every day. Know that we exist and only want the best for our kids, just as mothers do! For those fathers that are not actively in their children's lives, they should quickly realize what they mean to their kids. They should contact their children's mother and establish a co-parenting relationship - drive to their son or daughter's school to have lunch with them – BE MORE THAN JUST A FATHER. In my humble opinion, FATHERS ARE LIKE A$$#@LES, everybody has one - BUT NOT EVERYONE HAS A <u>DAD!</u> Don't let your kid(s) be in that FATHER category. I promise you, for every visit to a school, every phone call, every movie, every play-date, or games/recitals you attend – they will remember. I promise they will also remember the school plays you miss, the nights you don't call, the missed play-dates, and all the games and holidays that you're not there.

For those mothers who use their children as pawns and dangle them over the heads of the daddies who want to spend time with their kids, FEEL THANKFUL the father of your kids wants to be a dad! I say get over yourself and your ego and do something that facilitates a better co-parenting relationship. Tactfully stated, it doesn't pass the common sense test to punish or penalize your children for a failed relationship/marriage; especially, if their father has proven himself to be emotionally fit enough to positively influence their lives and has the potential/ability to provide for them. Removing a man like this from your children's lives is ridding them of one of the most important role-models they could ever have. In the end, the children are the ones who will suffer, and you'll read in this book how the effects can last for decades. You didn't get pregnant by yourself – if he's a MAN, don't block the blessings you or your kids are due to receive, and let him do his job!

This book contains stories of my fears before having children and practices that I employ as a dad today. I'm not perfect and will never claim to be, but since my kids were born, I have surrounded myself with MEN that take care of their responsibilities as a MAN and a dad! I seek counsel regularly from those who are objective, and I observe those who may not even realize they've helped me. From childhood to the present day – their teachings and influences are woven throughout the chapters of this book. **F|B**

Partners and Resources

I'd like to thank the select group of organizations below for educating me on their services and allowing me to create awareness of their existence to all who read this book. Navigating through challenging times like divorce and parental separation can be toxic for children -- I highly encourage you to seek out these organizations and others like them that are capable of
equipping you with co-parenting tools, counseling for children, and other related services.

Disclaimer: The personal views, opinions, and experiences in this book are
not necessarily those of the following organizations, and they are not liable for
any damage stemming from this publication.

New Hope Counseling Center - Kansas City, MO
816-340-6649
http://www.mynewhopecc.com

Mattie Rhodes Center - Kansas City, MO
816-471-2536
https://www.mattierhodes.org

America Family Law Center - Houston, TX
713-714-5100
https://www.americafamilylawcenter.org

Fathers for Equal Rights - Houston, TX
713-588-5870
http://www.fathersforequalrights4.org

Family Service Association - San Antonio, TX
210-299-2400
https://family-service.org

CenterPoint Counseling Center - Indianapolis, IN
317-252-5518
http://centerpointcounseling.org/

Memorial Child and Family Therapy - Houston, TX
832-794-2631
http://www.memorialchildandfamilytherapy.com

John Hopkins Medicine
(Behavioral Health) – Baltimore, MD
410-955-3599
https://www.hopkinsmedicine.org

Guardian House – San Antonio, TX
210-733-3349
https://guardianhouse.org/services/

Odyssey Family Counseling Center – Atlanta, GA
404-762-9190
http://www.odysseycounseling.org/programs-services...

Oakland Family Service – Oakland, CA
248-858-7766/ 877-742-8264
http://www.oaklandfamilyservices.org/

Denver Children Advocacy Center - Denver, CO
303-825-3850
https://www.denvercac.org

Avenues Counseling Center - St Louis, MO
314-529-1391
http://www.avenuescounselingcenter.org

Rubicon Family Counseling Services - Hartsville, SC
843-332-4156
http://www.rubiconsc.org

Center For Urban Families (Baltimore Responsible Fatherhood Project) – Baltimore, MD
410-367-5691
http://www.cfuf.org

Walk-In Counseling Center - Minneapolis, MN
http://www.walkin.org

The Family Institute (at Northwestern University) - Chicago, IL
847-733-4300
http://www.family-institute.org

ABOUT THE AUTHOR

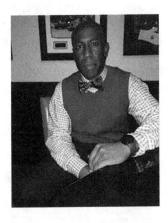

Anthonnie is a 41-year old, single dad of two children and a Lieutenant Colonel in the United States Army. Having grown up in Kansas City, Missouri, with both parents in the home, he observed first-hand how to be a dad, work hard, love your family, and the principle that things are earned, not given. That work ethic carried over into his academic studies as he earned a Bachelor of Science degree in Criminal Justice (Lincoln University - Missouri), a Masters degree in Business Administration (University of Phoenix) and a Masters degree in the Science of Strategic Intelligence (National Intelligence University – Defense Intelligence Agency). While serving our nation with distinction for over 18 years as an Army Officer, he took on single parent responsibilities five years ago, raising his 12-year old son while maintaining an active long-distance relationship with his nine year old daughter.

Through this journey of raising his son, Anthonnie encountered other men who obtained custody of their children, those who were fighting for custody, and those who lost hope of even spending quality time with their child due to a strained co-parenting relationship. He learned many things through these relationships, but nothing was more pressing than the counseling tools that are critical for children. He also learned that being an active parent with a child in a different state is challenging, but love and persistence make the difference. Having written multiple theses and led varying groups through decision making processes, Anthonnie journeyed into the world of published authors with the intent of telling his story, finding ways to equip and encourage other single dads to fight to be in their children's lives, and encourage single mothers to foster a respectable co-parenting relationship for the betterment of the children. Disclaimer: The personal views, opinions, and experiences in this book are not necessarily those of US Army and the Department of Defense, and they are not liable for any damage stemming from this publication.

CHAPTER 1 - BEING A DADDY: I WAS NOT READY

Despite the fact that my father worked 6-7 days a week as I was growing up, I was truly blessed to grow up in a household with two parents. I imagine that my mom felt like a single parent at times, but from my viewpoint, my dad's presence was felt ALL THE TIME. When he wasn't working, it was like GOD was home because he was trusted, respected, and feared. Throughout my life, as a boy, a teenager, and eventually a young adult, my father was always the man I feared the most but wanted desperately to be like. Of course, there were things I knew I could do better or different as a dad, but he embodied the core values every man should have. Growing up, I watched him love my mother and account for her shortfalls. He loved my sister and I in a way that only a Dad could, and he ensured that we were accountable for our actions. He was a provider and protector, and he ensured we had constant access to our heritage because the family name of my father and mother was important. At 18 years old, I was a young man who knew where his family came from because of all the lessons, stories, and inter-actions with the seniors in my family. I knew how to check the oil and tire pressure in my car. I knew how to establish a home bud-get, balance a check book, read utility statements, and pay bills. Above everything, I knew what hard work and dedication to family and friends was, and it was imperative that I do the same for mine when the time came.

Yes, my father did it right. He made being a daddy look easy, but I would be lying if I told you that I was ready to be a father in those first few hours after my wife (at the time) told me she thought she might be pregnant. Like lots of men, the first thing out of my mouth was the clumsy question, "How do you know?" The next thing out of my mouth was, "We need to get a more expensive pregnancy test!" I was nervous, and I damn sure wasn't happy! My wife being pregnant during this period of time in our lives was not a part of the plan. At the time, I was a young Captain in the US Army, and we were newlyweds and new homeowners with plans of enjoying time together before having children. For her, the results of the pregnancy test were welcomed, not for me, and I let it be known.

After the second pregnancy test, the discussion got heated between us, and we both had valid points. Abortion wasn't an option for her, but it certainly was for me. I admit, it wasn't my finest hour, and I could've gone about things differently. First and foremost, I was concerned that her chronic autoimmune disease (Lupus) would make delivering our child a high-risk pregnancy. Additionally, my mother suffers from Lupus, so I knew first-hand the problems it could cause. I was scared for my wife and our unborn child. Secondly, I was concerned about the brand new house we just purchased, my new job assignment, the cost of raising a child, and whether I was enough of a man to be a dad to a child. I vividly remember going to one of the many ultrasound appointments that seemed to always happen at the most inopportune times. I was extremely busy at work, and taking time away from that for an ultrasound was an encumbrance I could live without. Before I walked in the door, I was thinking to myself that I needed the doctor to finish quickly so I could get back to work. After being at the hospital for an hour, I grew more and more impatient. The doctor was doing all that was necessary for my wife and child, but I didn't care. She conveyed that she needed to run some additional tests. I said, "I have to get back to work; so, this needs to move faster!" The doctor and my wife looked at me with disgust! Yes, I was insensitive, thinking about taking care of the mission at work instead of caring about the tests being run for our future son. This was another hour I look back on and regret my actions and words. I had to understand things don't always happen when you want them to, and I had to get comfortable with the fact that having a child was going to happen.

So, what did I do? I do what I always do – consult with the people in my life that have been down the road I'm traveling. I was encouraged to have hope and pray often that my wife's illness wouldn't affect her nor our child. I was also reminded of my upbringing – the family and friends that shaped me into the man I was at that time. After getting beyond the anxiety, I welcomed the practical advice about parenting my family and friends knew we needed. As the pregnancy progressed, I can play back the things that were said to me that seemed obvious but ultimately became invaluable.

Papa Andrews: Get a gate for those stairs....

Dad: Start a 529 college fund and update that life insurance policy....

Robert Gerald: Be the most important role-model he sees everyday....

Maurice Reynolds: Teach him things he won't learn in school....

COL Ryan Janovic: Don't F--- this up....

All the advice and encouragement was certainly appreciated, but I still struggled. As a kid, I enjoyed spending time with cousins DJ and Dennis, but I had just as much fun spending time with both of my grandfathers. One was a Pastor in Kansas City, Missouri, with his own church, Morning Star Baptist Church, and the other – a devoted member at his church, Metropolitan Baptist Church, for over 35 years. Yes, they were old men who hung out with old people, but I was a bit of an old soul. I liked being in a church meeting in a suit just as much as I did playing kickball at recess. If I did watch cartoons, I preferred the rarely heard of cartoon called COPS over Winnie the Pooh because it was about adults fighting crime as opposed to a Bear who loved honey. Truth is, I was an impatient kid, and that didn't exactly change much by the time I earned a commission as a Second Lieutenant in the US Army.

Fast-forward some 11 years later – I'm a single dad who is still a bit impatient, but I'm quite fond of most kids and believe my own are the best gift GOD could give to a man. Moreover, I enjoy seeing parents interact with their kids, discipline their kids, brag on their kids, and mold their kids. When scrolling through my Facebook, I usually will hit "Like" on every post with a child and parent simply because I see the parallels and can identify with their journey. I absolutely LOVE my two beautiful children, and I am humbled that I have the opportunity to shape and mold two souls to be better than me in whatever endeavors they engage in.

For those who may already be traveling down this road or those who just became dads, I congratulate you and offer a few words of advice:

1. **Foster a REAL relationship with your Dad, a dad-like figure, a mentor, or close family member/friend who is a father:** Although I consult with my dad the most, I also consult with cousins, mentors, and close friends routinely for advice. Remember, advice doesn't always come in words – if you have a real relationship with this figure, you'll observe what "right" looks like.

2. **Turbulent times are inevitable, but a more seasoned dad can help guide your actions and decisions – LISTEN TO THEM.** In the end, you as a man are going to make your own decisions, but making an uninformed one could be a detriment to you and your children.

3. **Get past the idea that there will not be a perfect time and/or perfect conditions for you to be a dad.** There's nothing wrong with wanting your child to have more than you had growing up. However, having a child can serve as motivation to reach that next rung on the ladder (financially, spiritually, emotionally). Continuing to grow and identifying your weaknesses is a good thing so long as you're dedicated to fixing them.

4. **Focus on all the reasons why you would be a good dad, and acknowledge the things that you need to improve upon to be an even better Dad.** I would offer that having self-worth and the will to be as good (or better) a Dad than your own, is a true motivator. If you didn't have a Dad growing up, seek others in your same situation and remain focused on giving your child everything you didn't have. **F|B**

CHAPTER 2 - WHY DO KIDS NEED THEIR DAD

It wasn't until my son came to live with me that I realized how many strong mothers would argue that they raise their children better than the father could....I've heard it all!

.... A son will always have a closer connection with his mother....

.... It's not hard to teach him how to be a man....

.... I'll take her on play-dates so she knows how a man should treat a woman....

.... I got this......stay in your lane....

.... I can do everything for my kids that their father can do....

.... He needs a stable environment, only his mother can provide that....

The day I started writing this book was the day the following sentiments were expressed from someone I know: "our son is scared of you," "you don't have to discipline him that way," and "he needs his mother more than he needs you." Of course, I call BULL&^%$ on ALL of that ridiculous rhetoric, but it can be difficult trying to get someone to see something they don't want to see.

Later that night, I happened to be watching tv, and a short clip with action movie star Terry Crews on the show "The View". I can't say I listened much when the clip began, but what caught my attention were the words, "I can do everything for Evan that Jim can do for Evan". These were the words that were coming out of co-host Jenny McCarthy's mouth, and she was referring to Evan's father and star, actor Jim Carrey. I believe I understood what she was trying to say, but I don't think it came out the way she intended. Thankfully, actor Terry Crews, a guest on the show promoting a book about fatherhood, stood his ground. He stated, "There are things that you need from your father." He continued, "A father gives the child his/her name, protection, and confidence." While it appeared that McCarthy was proud of her son's attributes and her abilities as a mom, Crews' words, "kids need their fathers" resonated with me. At that moment, I began to reflect on what life would've been like without mine.

The reflection part wasn't hard. I watched my dad interact with his dad when I was a kid. I listened to my dad tell stories of life in the Eason household. I couldn't quite grasp the importance at the time, but the Eason name and the men that created the reputation of our family was important to my dad. He watched his dad serve GOD as a pastor in multiple Baptist churches for over 25 years. His uncles were business owners, Shriners, and dads themselves. Want to get my dad fired up? Mention the name EASON, and you'll hear him start talking about uncle Red's classy suits, uncle John's fuel station and car repair shop, or uncle Labon's Shriners parade for kids. Don't forget the caffeine because once he starts, he'll go on forever!

I didn't understand then, but today I understand and share his enthusiasm. I have more PRIDE in my family's name or brand than I do in other trendy brands. Do I own Air Jordans? Sure I do, but what I endorse by mouth, photos, or in written text has Team Eason associated with it – and I'm proud of that!

Crews also spoke about protection and how vital it is for a child. Fact is, when a father is deeply involved in his child's life, the by-product is confidence and strength. I'm not suggesting that my mother was less of a parent physically because she's actually two inches taller than my Dad. She taught me how to maintain a home, do laundry, cook for myself, and treat people with dignity and respect. All the things I do on a daily basis in my home for my kids, I owe to my mom!

On the other hand, my Dad was the provider, disciplinarian, and protector. My father working six or seven days a week represented financial security for our family. It meant the lights would stay on, our family would eat everyday, we would have a nice Christmas in the winter, a family vacation in the summer, and a few dollars left to put into a savings account. In order to achieve all that my dad wanted for our family, it meant I was getting Reeboks instead of Jordans for Christmas. It meant we were eating pork chops instead of steak, and the light damn well better be turned off if you weren't using it. In order to save money for vacations, we shopped at Aldi's instead of Price Chopper or Safeway for many items. I can appreciate it now, but I was an ungrateful kid at times. I wanted Jordans and British Knights, NOT Reeboks. I wanted a Starter jacket, NOT a Members Only jacket. I didn't see the big deal about the lights being on all the time – but obviously the electric bill didn't have my name on it. I wanted every vacation to be a seven day cruise, NOT Lake of the Ozarks! Bottom line, he afforded us a life with things that others didn't have. No, I didn't have a Starter jacket, but I went on a vacation every summer. No, I didn't have any Jordans, but there was money for me to attend college when I graduated high school. That's what a PROVIDER looks like to me!

In my household, my mom was quick to pull her belt out on my sister and I when we didn't behave or follow directions. Sometimes she'd use the belt – sometimes not. I was an arrogant kid with a big mouth who spoke his mind to my mom when I didn't like something. I knew where the line was, and I would test it with my mom because she was compassionate and caring. That was NEVER the case with my dad and discipline. Don't get me wrong, he was a very wise and generous man, but there was no mistaking that he was the "King of the Castle" as he would say. He was the "Lion in the Jungle" that you would tip-toe around and never make eye-contact with if you had done something wrong. He didn't tolerate my sister and I being disrespectful to my mother, and acting like a fool in school was a death sentence. My sister and I hated hearing the words, "Just wait till your daddy gets home!" These were literally the times when I didn't care that my dad was working six or seven days a week. In my father's house, my dad didn't need a belt! Him yelling at me was almost as bad as a belt – and his subtle movements in my direction were even worse. If you were wrong, the dimple in the middle of his nose would indicate you were about to have a bad day, week, or month. At times, I would run from my mom when she pulled her belt out or get on my knees and pray while she was looking – in hopes that it would keep my butt safe. Those tactics didn't work with my dad. At age ten, my sister stole a candy bar from a store, and as a result, my dad walked my sister into the store, returned the candy bar, and took her to the Police Station down the street.

This was beyond a leather belt. My dad spoke to the officer and requested that she be taken and told what would happen to her if she stole anything else in the future. If you did the crime, you were going to pay for it, PERIOD. Discipline came with everything we did, and he would reinforce the rules my mom set.

As a protector, he wasn't just physically stronger than my mother. He wasn't just the man who defended me in front of the neighbors who were older than me – he taught me how to protect myself in ways that go far beyond anything physical in nature. He showed me how to read the fine print on contracts, what a credit card interest rate is, how to conduct in-depth research on an item before I purchase it, and of course staying away from the wrong types women. As a teenager, I got myself into a predicament that could've cost me the very job I have today. After learning of the incident, my dad addressed the appropriate parties involved and protected me and our family name from future harm. In essence, many of the things that life has thrown at me, my Dad taught me how to protect myself from them.

So, yes, kids need their dads! In today's society, they are needed more than ever before. I can say this because of the people I've encountered as an adult who have and have not had their dad in their lives. Am I suggesting that kids don't take the wrong road at times while growing up? Not at all! As rigid as my household was, I still made mistakes, but I was afraid to see my dad afterwards. He was a deterrence for other things that I thought about doing but knew the consequence, and I didn't want to catch his wrath. During interviews with women for this book, a pattern surfaced regarding dating. Women indicated that not having a dad in their lives made them seek attention. The women I spoke with felt insecure in themselves, and they allowed themselves to be mistreated in relationships. Those with dads or dad-like figures, asserted they needed less attention, felt more confident, and only entertained men who treated them in ways their dads treated them. The men I spoke to indicated that not having a dad impacted their ability to remain committed in relationships. None of these things were shocking – we've all seen it before, but what was consistent across the males and females I spoke to for this book was the pride associated with the family name. Those who didn't have a dad in their lives admitted to reaching out to their fathers' family members or even private companies to learn the history of their family name. Seemingly, most of us yearn to know where we came from because that history tells a story and provides a bit of focus to improve or sustain ourselves and our family name. **F|B**

CHAPTER 3 - A MAN AND HIS SON: A DAY IN THE LIFE

The day I assumed physical custody of my son, was the day I transitioned to a daddy that emphasized the importance of discipline while being understanding and compassionate. The discipline part I knew I could do very easily. I was always the "bad cop" or "disciplinarian" in the house during our marriage. I grew up in a rigid household, had been in the Junior Reserve Officers Training Corps (JROTC) for four years in High School, the Senior Reserve Officer Training Corps (SROTC) for four years in College, and entered the US Army as a Second Lieutenant upon graduating from Lincoln University (Jefferson City, Missouri). Fast-forward 15 years to a Field Grade Officer in the US Army that possesses Obsessive Compulsive Disorder (OCD) tendencies. Admittedly, I am a neat freak who only stores shoes in closets, never goes to bed without washing the dishes and wiping down countertops, makes the bed immediately after getting out of it, and shops for groceries in a way that ensures the items in the grocery basket are bagged in an organized way. The understanding and compassionate part was new for me, and I wasn't afraid to admit it. Realizing that it was just him and me moving to Tampa, my initial solution was to find a psychologist for my son to help him emotionally deal with our divorce, as well as separation from his sister. The rest I would have to do on my own, one day at a time. I also knew I had to establish a routine in the house for predictability. Parents who've been around their kids will tell you how resilient their children are, but ask my son, DJ what he likes about living with daddy and he'll describe an environment where he knows what to expect – an environment that's predictable.

Our day-to-day grind....

0530 – Action: Wake up, personal hygiene and getting dressed prior to ensuring DJ is up. **Explanation:** Like most 12 year olds, he gets distracted very easily, therefore, my presence has to be within earshot. If not, he turns into a child body-builder in the mirror counting his muscles instead of brushing his teeth and getting dressed.

0600 – Action: Wake up DJ, prepare a light breakfast (breakfast bar, oatmeal, Milk),and begin "daddy overwatch."

Explanation: Some of you may laugh about "daddy overwatch," but during the first days of moving to Tampa in 2015, it was clear that I would never make it to work on time if I let him prepare for school on his own. "Daddy overwatch" consisted of me forcing DJ to move to the next step of his morning without delay. Subconsciously, I knew this would be the case because his mother would often complain about his lack of focus in the mornings when she would get him ready for school. This window of time is only 30-minutes, but I coin it "organized chaos." I'm saying things like "get out of bed, make that bed up quickly, keep your feet moving, your muscles aren't getting any bigger in the mirror, tie your shoes faster, chew that vitamin, hurry up and eat, brush your hair, get that back pack on," and "let's ride."

He's saying things like:

.... *I'm up....*

.... *I'm trying to make up my bed....*

.... *My feet are moving....*

.... *My muscles are getting bigger....*

.... *I'm tying them as fast as I can....*

.... *Why do I have to eat standing up....*

.... *My hair is longer than yours, it takes time....*

.... *I got my back pack....*

0630 – Action: Depart the house, drop DJ at "Before/After School Care", begin commuting to work.

Explanation: The trip to school from our home is a short one; literally three minutes and we're at the curb. I use the time wisely to get him in the right frame of mind for tests and discuss after school activities. The most important moment of the day approaches when I sign him in, and it's time for me to leave his school. As a Daddy who exchanges "I love you" many times a day with his son, I depart without kissing or hugging him. Yes, of course, he'd be embarrassed if I did such a thing in front of his friends. He is, however, more than ok with executing the Eason handshake, and I couldn't be more proud. That said, every kid is different; find what works best for you.

7:30a – 5:30p – Action: Work, plan, work, and plan **Explanation:** This is an extraordinary responsibility that I wanted and have been blessed by GOD to receive. From the time I drop him at school, to the time I pick him up, I'm thinking about a pediatrics appointment, his teeth, how much homework he's going to have, what I'm to cook for dinner, when's the next time we'll get to see my daughter Adri, when the next 5K that we'll run in is, what time the Chiefs game starts, what time the volunteer project starts next week, and how many Madden football video games we are going to play before he beats me.

5:45p – 7:45p Action: Pick up DJ from school/basketball practice,feed him a snack, check homework, cook, preparation activities for the next day.
Explanation: Upon my arrival to his school, I am able to read his body language instantly and determine if our evening is going to be a turbulent one. He's either knocking me down to tell me how great of a test score he earned or avoiding my questions about a test he didn't do so well on. What he doesn't know is, pass or fail, I'm pretty damn happy to see him! The ride home is fairly quick, but we usually discuss his day. After getting home, he gets the mail from the mailbox and starts his evening ritual. Similar to my tone in the morning, I'm pressing him in the evening and for good reason. Since he goes to bed around 8:45pm, moving around the house without meaningful action is wasting time we cannot get back.

That snack he eats is a quick one, the effort he puts in his homework is focused and deliberate, and I assist at every step to ensure he understands what he's doing. That said, there have been long nights. He attends a great school. Therefore, I expected there to be a challenging curriculum, but I don't remember crafting paragraph summaries from reading assignments in the 2nd grade, division math problems in the 3rd grade, and cycles of metamorphosis

in the 4th grade. The 5th and 6th mixed grade fractions and tec-
tonic plates took me a minute, but I figured out how to check to
ensure I was able to reinforce the lesson plan, thanks to Google!
After completing his homework, he takes a bath and prepares his
clothes for the next day. Dinner follows these actions so there's no
compassion from me. The shower is a thorough yet succinct one
– "scrub and rinse everything three times – don't play – turn my
water off!" Next, his school uniform gets laid out for school; shirt,
shorts/pants, socks, and shoes. I tell him "details are important"
so he understands that small things like loosening his shoe laces,
unbuttoning his shirt and placing the belt through the loops the
night before saves time in the mornings. At 8 pm, dinner is served!
I keep it simple, but vary the meals. He's not a big fan of veggies,
but if they're sweet he'll eat them -- glazed carrots, cream style
corn, and sweet peas with turkey bacon. Shrimp, salmon, turkey
meatballs, and chicken are his favorite meats, but chili and Jiffy
cornbread are also a must. While eating dinner, he talks to his
mom and Adri on the phone. I try to be patient while he talks to
his mom, but as soon as Adriana comes to the phone, I'm usually
interfering with the conversation. After dinner, we say the Lord's
Prayer, and spend a few minutes talking about life as he sees it
(politics, family, favorite gym shoes, video games, academics, and
girls), and then it's bed time.

From the time my alarm clock goes off in the morning, just
about every action has a purpose. My methods may be different
from others, but they are necessary. Meaning, my son didn't start
out eating breakfast standing up, but after two weeks of watching
him daydream while eating, an adjustment had to be made. He initially saw standing up as punishment, but later realized it was for
the best, and he began to have fun with it. Another example would
be the issue he took with preparing his clothes for school the night
prior. His mom used to do this for him, and the detail I directed it
to be done in was foreign. My answer to this was to show him the
clock when he began getting dressed after preparing his clothes
his way. A week later we timed him getting dressed after preparing his clothes in a more detailed manner. He found that he wast-
ed so much time trying get the knots out of his shoes, unbuttoning his shirts and pants and putting on the belt, that he couldn't
argue with the results. On the surface these things are practical
and appear to only facilitate us getting out of the house in a time-

ly manner. What lies beneath the surface, however, are principles (time management, attention to detail) he learned that eventually he'll use routinely as a high school or college student and a working professional. **F|B**

CHAPTER 4 - A PROMISE TO MY PRINCESS

I had been a daddy for three years, I'd changed several of DJs stinky diapers, and taken a few family trips when my wife talked about trying to have a girl. I still had concerns about her health and the health of the baby, but being a dad to a second child wasn't going to be nearly as tough as the first. Upon learning that we were having a girl, a feeling of pride and uncertainty came over me. Pride in what I could teach her-- how to change the oil in her car, invest her money wisely, and take her on daddy-daughter dates. The uncertainty stemmed from trivial things from having to do her hair to my fears of her being pushed to the ground by a bully at school or dumped by a boyfriend. All in all, when Adriana came along, I was ready. Like most daddies, my thinking was that my little girl could do no wrong. Of course, that was in the early stages before she began to take on an identity and develop a personality. That personality can be deceiving. If you know her, you've seen her timid ways around people, but realize she is lurking in the shadows doing stuff she's not supposed to be doing. When she's caught for doing something wrong, she finds a place to stare at in the ceiling (or the clouds) and holds it until she's no longer in trouble. Of course, all kids have something they do that doesn't make sense – this one belongs to her. Despite that, she makes it easy for me to be her dad because she respects and understands my rules when she's with me, and she even listens and follows directions better than her brother.

The true test for me and most dads is refraining from playing the favoritism game with my daughter and being the same disciplinarian with her as I am with my son. It took time, but a number of women I trust, conveyed that the same approach I've taken with my son has to be the same with my daughter. It's definitely easier said than done because she lives with my ex-wife in a different state, and I prefer to spend my time spoiling her, watching her show me a new dance, and listening to her talk about her day. However, there have been times where I've had to punish her from a distance. When I facetime her and her room was repeatedly found messy or she was failing to turn in her homework, I suspended her iPhone access. I hated to do it, but I realized I would be crippling my daughter by coddling her at times when discipline is required. Routine things I always tell her:

.... Saying thank you to whomever prepared the meal she's about to eat....

.... Praying before eating....

.... Making up your bed when you get up....

.... Clean the current area before going to play in a different one....

.... Be nice to people....

Yes, these things are common, but the message builds and the meanings evolve into life lessons I must teach her each year she gets older. Although she doesn't live with me, my daughter knows she can talk to me about anything, and she will never be punished for telling the truth. She'll have undivided attention at bedtime, and her bedroom in my home will always belong to her and only her. She knows I'll be there to pick her up when she falls off of her hover board. I'll be there for that first breakup in high school. My presence will be felt when she gets that "D" in statistics and the "A" in science. We'll celebrate her first paycheck. As often as possible, she'll be exposed to the world and the many cultures within it. I'll be there to point out the good, bad, and ugly on her first house. No matter what it is – she knows daddy is always going to be here.

F|B

CHAPTER 5 - POSITIVE INFLUENCES: FIND THEM

The old saying "It takes a village to raise child" was something my parents believed in greatly. My parents were excited about the fact that my elementary school principal (Ms. Grant) would pull a disruptive student into her office and spank them with one of her paddles without hesitation. As an eight year old, I tried the system and lost when I acted out on the playground one day and got into a fight. Ms. Grant swung the paddle three times and connected three times; then she called my parents. While I'll never forget Ms. Grant, there were many others that my parents exposed me to growing up. Police officers, political officials, business owners, teachers, bus drivers, plant workers and railroad trainmasters were all influential in some way or another. The biggest take-away for me was that success didn't come easy, and all of them worked hard to be successful and provide for their families.

As a parent striving to do the same for my children, it's important that everyone understands the people I idolized the most were my parents. I didn't realize it at the time, but my sister and I were being groomed for life. I take nothing away from my mom whatsoever – she taught my sister and I how to be independent at age 10 or 11 years old. Doing laundry, washing dishes, cleaning floors, and taking out trash, were things I hated. It wasn't until I arrived at college and observed that an alarming number of people in the dormitory didn't know how to do laundry and lived like pigs because they weren't required to clean and do laundry at home. The monumental lessons, however, were taught (age 11) when my dad would sit my sister and I down and showed us how to read water, electric, and gas bills. The next time he'd show us auto insurance, mortgage, and credit card bills. The next time he'd show us how to read bank statements and balance a check book. Too much for a kid, right? No, I'd say I was among a small number of freshmen in my dorm that knew how to write a check, balance a check book, and pay my own auto insurance bill.

My dad illustrated how an annual salary of $14,000 wasn't going to buy a big house or a luxury car. After taxes, social security, the mortgage, car payments, the utilities (water, electric, phone, basic cable), life and medical insurance policy premiums, car fuel, groceries, saving account deposit, and 401K deposit, there would be little left to go out on a Friday night with friends. Of course, as I was being taught all of this, I would push back and say things like, "I'll keep the lights turned off" – his response would be, "What about heat in the winter and A/C in the summer?" "Ok, well, I don't really need a life insurance policy, and I'll just pay the medical bill IF I have to go to the hospital." He laughed! "Do you know what a visit to the emergency room costs? –you're better off just paying the monthly insurance premium so you don't have to pay for the entire emergency room bill!" Determined not to let him win, I said, "The savings account isn't really a need – I can work without that." His response was, "Ok, don't put money into it, but when you get a flat tire or two and you don't have a fund for emergencies, don't say I didn't warn you."

I vividly remember being 18 years old and preparing to leave for college in a couple of days. My parents and I were doing some last minute shopping for my dorm room and stopped at a gas station before going home. While there, my dad asked, "Did you get your fluids and tires checked yesterday?" I replied, "Huh?" I meant no, I just didn't want to say it aloud. Needless to say, he went from 0 to 100 really quickly! "You're leaving for college in less than two days – have a 2.5 hour drive, and you haven't even checked the oil or the tire pressure?!" He continued, "What are you thinking son, you don't drive for 2.5 hours without checking your car out, and you know that." I didn't think it was that bad; it wasn't an eight hour drive, but he was angry—really angry. After that, I wanted nothing more than to leave my parents' house, but I missed the lesson he always tried to teach my sister and I from years past. As a parent today, I now understand that getting my fluids and tires checked wasn't so much about the drive. To paraphrase his many years of lectures, it was clear that BEING PREPARED (in principle) and HAVING A PLAN would facilitate success. Ultimately it makes life easier personally and facilitates success professionally.

At 41 years old, with two children of my own and physical custody of my son, it's been one of my highest priorities to give my kids what my parents gave me – an opportunity to meet, interact with, and learn from positive people I consider role-models. My son holds both of his grandpas in high regard and loves spending time with his uncles (DJ and Dennis) because laughter is imminent. Beyond that, the village I surround him with is deliberate. DJ's dentist, my neighbor and owner of her own dentistry for over 11 years, has been a great role model for both of my kids. A child psychologist and business owners are also among the number of women role models involved in my kids' lives.

My son first met Robert Ray (aka Dr. Rob) over the phone when I called to seek advice when DJ was sick a few months after we arrived in Tampa. An emergency room doctor whom I've had a close relationship with for over 20 years answered the call one night when I had questions about children's cold medicine and Vapor Rub. For years I had been following an old method of using the vapor rub and bundling up. Doctor Rob gave me advice to the contrary – "Leave the shirt off after you put the Vapor Rub on him and put him to bed." he said. I followed his advice, and the next morning DJ said, "who is Dr. Rob? -- He must know what he's talking about. I can finally breathe." A few months later, Dr. Rob came to visit for a weekend, and of course, I had planned to show him my town. However, from the minute he landed and met DJ, he began to impress upon him the importance of hard work and dedication. There were discussions about being a military service member or a doctor, and how doing well in school now will translate to success later. I couldn't have been happier – here was another man that wasn't his father, providing him with insight. One day, I know that this will give him confidence, knowing someone he knows has already been down the road he's traveling. Unfortunately, but fortunately, I did not show Dr. Rob my town. He literally spent the whole weekend teaching DJ moves with the Kappa Kane, eating junk food with him, and playing pool and video games. In DJ's words, "We had an EPIC weekend with Dr. Rob. He should come back next weekend."

Lieutenant Colonel Rob Gerald (aka Uncle Rob) is another close friend (of 17 years) and role model that has taught DJ life lessons. Uncle Rob has reinforced my lessons of knowing your priorities and taking care of them ahead of anything else. During my time in Tampa, the Army called, and travel abroad was required. Uncle Rob opened his doors and family to DJ. Beyond that, he and his family have always been there regardless of where the Army has assigned us. He didn't just give my son a place to sleep but also a home that embodies values, love, manhood, and fatherhood. On the back end of a trip, DJ will tell you he ate good and tried hard to beat Uncle Rob at video games – which is great. I know his week was also spent doing pushups, homework, and learning about military academies. I know that Mr. Rob's favorite quote, <u>"Do what you have to do – so you can do what you want to do"</u> resonated with DJ every day after school. And during summer trips to Las Vagas and Hawaii to visit Dr Rob and Uncle Rob, these men treat my daughter as if she was their own. Sounds too good to be true....probably....not everyone your kid(s) spend time with will be perfectly aligned with your same parenting preferences. I'm lucky in that what happens at Mr. Rob's home happens at my home. DJs expectation is that his homework comes before playing video games, and chores come before watching tv. He expects to run 3 miles with me on a Saturday before going to the movies, bowling, gun range, shooting pool or to the go cart track.

As parents, we often worry about the negative encounters our kid(s) may have at school, on the street, and on the internet. Most parents would speak with the teacher about problems at school and take steps to restrict their kids from sites on the internet. These actions are certainly proper, but I'd offer that soliciting the help of the individual outside the home to reinforce your message can be monumental. Imagine what the long-term effects could be if your child spent one or two hours a month being influenced by a righteous figure? Find that teacher, welder, coach, military service member, doctor, or entrepreneur and leverage that resource to spend time with your kids. Men – if you're the righteous figure I just described, I encourage you to refrain from turning a blind eye to situations in which you know a person of your caliber can be a positive influence. I encourage you to take the time to help mold the youth of the future. **F|B**

CHAPTER 6 - LIVING WHAT YOU TEACH

You've heard the stories or lived it in your home as a kid – "Do what I say, not as I do!" Yep – those are the words your parents would routinely say. Growing up, I wasn't allowed to curse, but that didn't stop my parents from doing it. My sister and I could easily get four days of punishment for not completing chores properly. Seemingly, you would think it meant my parents would keep the house immaculate when my sister and I were away. Nope – not a chance! Trash would pile up, dishes would go unwashed, rooms wouldn't get vacuumed and laundry would sit. As a teenager and then as a young adult it made me MAD to think I could get in trouble for emulating my parent's actions. In the grand scheme of things, these things I lived with are a bit trivial, but what if my parents partied a lot and had problems getting to work on time? Could they, in good conscience, threaten me with punishment if I didn't do my chores before going outside to play? If my parents failed to pay the electric bill on-time because they spent the money at the casino, could they punish me for ditching school and having poor grades? Obviously, there are reasonable limitations since parents are parents and kids are kids, but the point is – parents owe it to their kids to live the same life expected of their kids.

In a home with two parents, this concept is much easier since only one parent has to be an example in the area the child should emulate. For those single dads and mothers, this may create a real lifestyle change. As previously stated, I have a small ounce of OCD, so there wasn't much of a lifestyle change in the area of structure and organization. Their shoes will never be found anywhere in the house other than their closet because that's the proper place for them. Dirty clothes always belong in a hamper; not on the floor. Clothes are properly folded or hung and stored with like articles of clothing. Waking up in the morning means your bed gets made up before doing anything else. Dirty dishes belong in the sink – not left on the table. All of these things and more are what I require but make no mistake – I follow my own rules. When showing my kids how to organize drawers and closets, I started in my room. I say to them "Pull out any drawer and open the closet door." They didn't understand at first, but after putting away clothes of their own, it became very clear what I expected. Some parents may argue this is too much for kids under 12 years old – I'd argue that's nonsense because it happens every day in my house. Does my son meet the mark every other week when it is time to do laundry? No! When I go to inspect his drawers, do I find them in disarray? Sometimes, Yes! Does Adri always get her shirts folded exactly right? No, not always! Are collared shirts hung in the closet with v-neck t-shirts? Absolutely, they are! However, what's clear is they know there's a STANDARD because I vocalize it daily, and they can also walk into my room and see the STANDARD for themselves.

Living what you teach certainly extends far beyond folding clothes – it's a reflection of "life" things as well. Meaning, a parent's actions in a grocery store with the check-out clerk should be aligned with how they expect their children to treat others. I once observed a disgruntled mother making life miserable for a cashier over a price check; then subsequently cursed her son out in the parking lot for being disrespectful to his teacher in class. Those who know me well will usually wait for my eyes to turn red when a double standard surfaces. This was definitely one of those times, but it wasn't my problem to handle. That said, if one of my children had responded by saying they thought it was okay to talk to people in this manner, I couldn't fault them. The young man in the store may or may not have done the same thing, but it was obvious to me that the cashier ringing up the groceries wasn't at fault for the price of the item. Being able to see yourself and your shortcomings isn't an easy thing, but it's senseless to think your children will conduct themselves differently than what you show them.

I agree it's a bit of a double edged sword because we as grown parents sacrifice a lot to provide for our children. You want to live life without a filter – without an authoritative figure- and live a fun lifestyle. I get it – but I'd offer that you gave that up when you had children, and therefore, you owe them your best self and your best example. Growing up, I watched my dad not only work hard but study for tests that facilitated promotion to new positions and higher pay at the railroad. I watched him put money into a savings account and purchase savings bonds each month. He could've easily used the money he spent on life insurance policies to buy a toy for himself or a ring for my mom, but he saw the importance of our family having a comfortable life should he pass on before us. He didn't just talk about it, he showed my sister and I how it was done, and I could see those sacrifices manifest themselves in short and long stretches of time. Those promotions he worked hard for led to savings bonds that helped pay for my college education. My dad isn't perfect – he knows it, and so do I. However, he equipped me with the tools and the lessons to be better than him, and now I pay it forward so that my children are better than me. **F|B**

CHAPTER 7 - SOMEONE ELSE'S JOURNEY

MAKING HIM A MAN

When I met her, I thought she was the one! She was beautiful, sexy, smart, caring, and family oriented – basically, all I wanted in a woman! As time went on, we built wealth, accumulated assets, and most importantly, we had a son. After my son was born, the negative attributes I ignored before began to manifest themselves, but I wasn't a quitter and fought to make my marriage work. Session after session, argument after argument, and sacrifice after sacrifice – we both fought for the marriage until we no longer could. What happened afterwards was a whirlwind that I'd like to forget, but it's impossible to let the memories go. Our divorce was brutal, like most of us that have gone through one, but that was a cake walk compared to what happened after the divorce was final. Yep, my son became a pawn! The signed arrangement we made was simple and equitable, but she found ways to skirt it and even ignore it.

Additionally, she found ways to keep him from me, and many times she refused to even have discussions about simple things like picking him up/dropping him off. Any discussion of him coming to live with me full time only infuriated her. When his grades suffered, she blamed me as if I was with him full time. She only communicated with me when child support was involved versus when he struggled emotionally. It's not hard to see that she allowed her anger from the divorce to get in the way of us co-parenting. She would often speak as if I was incapable of raising our teenage son. Now I'm not rich, but I am an educated professional with financial stability. Additionally, I am emotionally and spiritually fit. Most importantly, I possess a strong support system for my son and a strong desire to raise my son and give him the tools to be a better man than me.

As you read my story, it may come across as if she is the only one to blame. She's not. When this all began, I didn't have all the tools to be a good husband! I dated women for the wrong reasons and could easily move on to the next one. Courtship was foreign to me, and I attracted women who didn't demand it. These lessons and a number of others weren't taught to me by my dad. He was a rigid man who provided for our family, and I appreciated that tremendously. That said, he lacked compassion, wasn't present for important moments in my life, and didn't give me tools to make better decisions regarding women. As a result, I gravitated to my amazing mother, but it didn't exactly make up for what I needed from my dad. Bottom line, I married a woman I was in love with on paper. That wasn't enough to make our marriage last.

I'll own my part for marrying someone I didn't love, but raising a son is a separate matter. The relationship I had with my wonderful mother is one that I've had with no other person on earth. Therefore, I would never say my son doesn't need his mother. However, my dad left me to learn life's lessons on my own. I DIDN'T WANT THAT FOR MY SON! Sure, I had taken him to Hawaii, the Caribbean, Mexico, Jamaica, and many other places that I didn't travel to until adulthood, but those environments aren't the places where real life happens. He needed me on a daily basis, and I didn't believe I should have to fight his mother to be a constant figure in his life. I yearned to sharpen his shaving skills, improve his appetite for academics, and show him how to change the oil in my car. If it's not obvious, I was poised to make my son A MAN much earlier in his life.

Giving credit where its due, my Ex-wife came to realize late in his teenage years that she needed to love our son more than she hates me and sent our son to live with me. I AM GRATEFUL FOR THAT!!

Lastly, I say to all dads in this situation, don't tire or take a knee – your kid(s) need you to fight for them. To the mothers in a similar situation—wear this shoe if it fits, and give your kid(s) life by allowing their dad to play a major role. F|B

                                        - J Kevin, Washington, D.C.

A LITTLE GIRL'S DREAM

At 10 years old, life was normal for me and my family in Colorado. My mom would cook, take care of the house, and take care of me. My dad worked a lot, but even when he wasn't physically present, I always pictured him at home around the house and routinely heard his voice. Obviously, I loved my mom, but I was a daddy's girl and never envisioned life without him. At 14, things took a turn for the worst, and my parents divorced. To say it was life changing would be an understatement! Simply put, my dad moving out of our house crushed me as I couldn't help but wonder why this was happening, and what did I do to cause it? The more I asked my mom about my dad, the further away I was pushed from the truth and a relationship with him. One day led to the next and before I knew it, life was happening without my dad. In that same breath, it hurt me to the core to hear my mother say bad things about my dad.

Being 15 years old and starting high school was a whirlwind. During this time, my proms, family dinners and many other things occurred without my dad. Life's challenges as a teenager and high school student began to present themselves in ways that only my dad could help with. Things like building my confidence by knowing where my family name came from and teaching me the follow-through mechanics of my jump shot. I wanted and needed him, but I constantly wondered if he still cared about me. I remembered daddy - daughter dates as a little girl, but none as a teenager prior to my first date. Even more so, I just wanted my dad to do normal things with me aside from sending Christmas gifts or money for my birthday.

After graduating high school, I wanted a life with my dad, but I didn't know how because so much time had passed. At age 24, he reached out to me, and I learned that my mom decided it was best for her to run my dad out of our lives because their marriage didn't work out. What's worse is - he gave in to her demands!

Was I angry? - ABSOULTELY! It took some time to get over the fact that I've lived years without him as child and young adult. I've been married and divorced without him, I've started a great career without him, and I've became an avid sports fan without him. All things NO DAUGHTER SHOULD HAVE TO SHOULDER OR EXPERIENCE LIFE WITHOUT HER DAD! My life today is vastly different as I've channeled my emotions towards making everyday count with my dad. Don't get me wrong, I thank my mother for all she did to raise me, but days will past without me communicating with her. On the other hand, there isn't a day that goes by in which I don't communicate with my dad. He comes to my office for lunch, we run often, attend sporting events together and he gives me the love and support only he can give.

He's the voice of reason in my head and the person I vent to when a date didn't go well. My dream has been realized, and I'm thankful and hopeful that dads understand the value they can bring to a child's life. In that same breath, I'd offer that a mother who deters, prevents, or blocks her child(ren) from a capable father is guilty of their child's future downfalls. F|B

- Robyn, California

WE DIDN'T MAKE IT, BUT OUR SON WILL

I come from a close-knit family with two sisters and a brother. We've always been close, but each one of us has a unique relationship with my mom. What's always been missing is my biological dad. Growing up, I used to be confused about their relationship and his lack of presence in my life. I knew he wasn't physically too far, lived in the same community of other relatives, where I attended church and even hung out with my half-brothers, but we rarely connected! Little did I know, those experiences would prepare me for life as a mother and certain decisions I made to facilitate a relationship with my son's father.

Shortly after completing college, I met an amazing man who entered my life at the right time. It was fun and spontaneous, yet we were both young and really didn't think about the future. The turbulence started when I discovered I was pregnant, and his response was nothing at all like I expected. I mean, I wasn't looking for a proposal of marriage, but at the very least, I expected his words, "I will support you in whatever you decide." to be at least his bond.

The silver lining of it all was our son, but the strain from our relationship made co-parenting difficult to say the least. He was frustrated, and I was bitter, hurt, and still confused, especially because I knew his history of being raised by his uncle not his Dad! He was initially avoidant and unsure of what type of arrangement he wanted to be set up.........and I wanted GOD to touch his heart & make him the best father for our son. My model being a physically present (emotionally absent) Dad (stepfather) for over 20 years, I knew that wasn't an option for us (I really didn't want just that anyways), I stepped back and let GOD be GOD.

For a few years we fought about significant issues and petty ones, but in 2005, a revelation from not having my father at certain points during my childhood changed that. My personal growth and unconditional love I have for my son led me to the realization that he needs his father, and I needed to do my part to facilitate that. As dedicated as I had been as a mother, there were certain things only his dad could teach him. In essence, I/we chose our son, and all three of our lives changed for the better. The current arrangement as it relates to visitation has only improved over the years as we now live in the same region and increased time can be spent together (at a lower cost?) during school breaks, holiday breaks, special birthdays, music competitions, etc.

When it comes to child support, we have kept the amount relatively the same with a recent increase to cover half of car insurance! Our son was given a debit card managed by his father in 8th grade and extras are sent directly to him. Activity Fees, cost for summer camps and other activities are usually spilt down the middle. I consult with my son's father on all matters having to do with our son's well-being, and he consults with me - and there's genuine respect between the two of us. The result – our son knows how to maneuver in a single parent household as well as stand proudly in his role as big brother in a two parent household (he's blessed with the best Bonus Mom for him). He's achieved an independent relationship with GOD, pride in himself, knowledge that he is loved in a variety of ways by his parents and the ability to balance different rules/routines in two households. He's polite and respectful!

He carries a 3.8 GPA and is a committed leader in the band program, growing tennis player and well rounded young man! Most importantly he's received multiple college offers and he's poised to attend a HBCU with an academic scholarship and band scholarship.

For any woman reading my story, it's critically important that you choose your children and don't block the blessings that come with them spending time with their dad! KIDS NEED THEIR DAD! F|B

Marie, Illinois

THE MESSAGE: A FATHER OF THREE

There's no greater thing IN LIFE than that of a man being a dad to his children. Dads, allow that to sink in.........................from conception, you literally have the honor and responsibility to mold a brand new human being of your flesh and blood into an art teacher, railroad engineer, judge, dentist, entrepreneur, or renowned entertainer.

Life growing up with my father was good. He worked hard, had his own business and provided for my mom and me. He taught me how to be a man of the community, carry myself with pride and honor, and keep God first and foremost in my life. I saw him love my mother and care for her. I always imagined myself growing up to be just like my dad.

During my last year in college, I received a phone call and was informed that a young lady I slept with was pregnant. At the time, my mind was focused only on my new job, which was to start in 5 months. I didn't know what to do, or think, but felt that this was a set-up. I blamed her for getting pregnant, as if I had nothing to do in the matter. She had her own issues. It was a powder keg. After going through court appearance after court appearance, I was left bitter.

Eight years later I got married at the age 30. I think I was trying to be the man my dad was. I may have rushed things and attempted to force my life into my father's mold. From that marriage, a son was born. My son was what I wanted! I wanted to create for him in same ways my Dad created for me. However, his mom came from a different style of upbringing, and we clashed all the time. Soon after, I filed for divorce, and the war of custody began. Going through the divorce proceedings was hard. The temporary child support order was breaking me. I barely had enough to pay bills that we accumulated together; but that's what I was left with. I was not willing to concede the rights of my son. But God! My lawyer did something amazing! At the final court hearing, it appeared that a joint order would be put in place. My lawyer's closing statement was not to the judge, but to my ex-wife and I, as parents. She stated that she knew both of us loved our son with all our hearts and that he needed both of us. Both of us had good jobs; so there was no need for us to handicap the other to be a good parent. We both agreed that we couldn't work as a couple, but we would give our lives making sure our son had a chance. Custody was made joint, with us splitting education and healthcare.

Even though that worked out, I was still broken and felt like a failure. That's the perfect time for satan to attack. I, once again, was going down the road of trying to create an image that I had it all together . I was lost. I met someone else, much younger than me. We were ill suited for each other, and the relationship did not work out for long. Of course, another child was born. I was terrified, and initially, ashamed. However, what I saw as failure, was actually God telling me that he loved me. The birth of my daughter changed me. She has been with me since day one. She became my peace. She grounded me. I no longer longed for fantasy life. I just wanted to be a good dad to this little girl who adored me.

I met yet another woman when my daughter was about a year old. We married one year later, and have been together now for 14 years.

The phenomena that mothers not allowing dads to play a major role is alarming to say the least. Dads must understand that Real Eyes Realize Real Lies, and therefore, as men we must accept ALL responsibility for the lives we create.

In closing, I'd like to reiterate what being a dad is a blessing from God......There's no army known to man that could keep me from my kids. Truth in lending, my relationship with my oldest daughter has come with challenges – not a day that goes by that I don't wonder how to bridge the gap between us. As for my other two children, I interact with them every day in an effort to help them navigate through life as athletes and students in their respective high school and college programs. My son will graduate in December 2018 from Lincoln University (Missouri) with a 3.2 GPA and honors and will begin his career in Virginia Beach in March 2019. My youngest daughter carries a 4.0 GPA and plays Volleyball and Basketball.They've all made me a proud dad! F|B

Dennis, Illinois

CHAPTER 8 - CO-PARENTING: ARE YOU?

Emails and texts with no response, no returned phone or video calls, disregard for the terms of the divorce decree and informal agreements, displayed bitterness years after divorce, double standards and beyond. You name it, and I've likely encountered it or know multiple others who have. While I could write a book speculating about childhood or relationship/marriage woes as reasons, none of them warrant blocking an upstanding dad from his FLESH AND BLOOD! To each of you that are frustrated and feel like you have no options, I say REMAIN COMPOSED, KEEP TRYING TO COMMUNICATE WITH YOUR KID(S), and DOCUMENT YOUR EFFORTS with dates and times for EVERYTHING YOU DO! In essence, quitting and/or acting erratic is what she wants you to do, so don't give her the satisfaction. That said, I make no promises that these actions will keep the mother of your kids from being difficult, so prepare yourself. Things that are factual, written, recorded, etc. will all of sudden, not be factual – will not be what is written – will not be what is plain to hear or see. Yep, I'm suggesting that so long as she is angry and bitter, facts will not be seen as truth to her. Since my situation is a bit unique, and my ex-wife and I have joint custody of our two children, I'll be the first to admit that the right side of my brain wants to use her tactics and treat her in the same manner in which she treats me. The left side of my brain says THAT'S FOOLISH, stay on the right side of the line, and FOCUS ON THE KIDS!

Those who know me will tell you that raising my kids in the best possible environment is paramount! Hiding or avoiding issues about my son, depriving my son of time with his mom, and saying negative things about her in his presence would make me no better than her. Moreover, I'm a true believer that kids need to have both parents in their lives, and I'd be hurting my son by trying to put myself or any other woman in her place as their mother. For those of you walking down the same path, I'd invite you to take weekly pictures of the children for her awareness, encourage videocalls often, encourage and facilitate interaction with the children's teachers, dentist, counselor, and pediatrician. Be transparent and keep no secrets – I guarantee, your children will divulge them in due time. That said, I offer the following:

1.) **If divorce or a break-up is truly necessary, do all you can to foster a respectable relationship with the mother of the child.** Making a child takes two people, and the child didn't ask to be here. It's vitally important that you step up and ensure the mother of the child understands the important role you play in the child's life. Never forget that your kids are watching – do your best to have cordial conversations with their mother, and don't allow your ego to get in the way. Arguing in front of your children is setting the wrong example. Talking bad about the other parent in their absence isn't much better. This is easier said than done, but your kid(s) must see NO-SPACE on the parenting front – at least until they're mature enough to understand the circumstances revolving around the divorce or breakup.

2. **Seek co-parenting programs.** It only takes one parent possessing a big ego in a co-parenting relationship to impede progress. At the time of my divorce, my ex-wife and I sought counseling, but it was primarily to figure out if our marriage was really over. Did it work? No! Was it a waste of time? No – but I feel that we should've put our efforts into a co-parenting program like "New Day" at Centerpoint Counseling Center in Indianapolis or "H.O.P.E" at the Guardian House in San Antonio. Perhaps, having a non-biased individual (or team) with experience, practical exercises, solutions, and other related services to help us see ourselves as co-parents and a couple, may have gotten us off on the right foot. As time has gone on, and I'm smarter about what it takes to co-parent; I'm smarter about egos and how they can lead to arguments and I'm certain that one parent can't do it alone. Newsflash – if you're not co-parenting, you're hurting the child more than you are the other parent.

3. **Unless you're a child psychologist or marriage counselor – seek help for your children.** In certain circles and cultures in America, seeking professional help is frowned upon. Before 2010, I was one of those people, but I've wised up and now I say it's critically important. Don't help yourself get through a tough divorce by seeking professional help then turn into something you're not when it's time for your child to see a professional! The secret is changing the narrative with kids so they understand there's goodness in seeing a "kid helper" not a child psychologist. Upon my move to Tampa in 2014, I knew I needed a female "kid helper" to assist my son in coping with the divorce and with being away from his mom and his sister. Speaking from experience, DJ's time with her has been incredibly enlightening and productive. He says what he feels (topics: Mom, Dad, discipline, girls, homework, chores, puberty, etc) to someone that's not his parents which improved his level of confidence. His views/opinions helped me be a better dad. Adriana is not excluded from these sessions during her visits. She's benefited greatly, as the topics range from favorite subjects in school to mommy and daddy being apart and dating other people.

4. **Dads - Don't allow the fact that you live in a different state be the reason you don't have a relationship with your kid(s).** I'm not going to sugar coat this point – it is tough but not impossible. The geographical limitations can be frustrating and the mother of your kid(s) may be difficult to deal with. However, your obligation is to your children NOT the mother; so fight to be their dad everyday if necessary. When two parents have different styles of discipline, different diets, and different ways of dealing with problems, you must possess a never-quit attitude and fight to remain in your child's life. Call/videocall throughout the week, contact teachers, counselors, principals, physicians, dentists, etc as often as possible to check on your children. Simply put, these people provide a service and/or care to your FLESH AND BLOOD, and therefore, they should know who you are and vice versa.

5. **NO SECRETS**. I can't stress the point enough that directing your children to keep secrets from their mom sets a bad precedence in the short term and creates major problems long term. DON'T DO IT! When children realize a situation is bad, and you as the parent attach "a secret" to it, a divide is created between you and the other parent. Unfortunately, it won't stop there! Once you establish this as precedence, you can expect your children to begin keeping secrets for things they do at home and school which ultimately decreases the open and honest dialogue between you and the child. In short, be responsible enough to communicate with the other parent so you don't have to tell your child to keep secrets!

A person I trust stressed to me a few weeks ago that REAL EYES REALIZE REAL LIES (R.E.R.R.L)! Telling your children lies about the other parent may work in the short term, but by age 10 or 11, they'll eventually REALIZE the LIES you're telling. Like most kids, my kids question things, and when they're ready, they ask hard questions. What's interesting is when their mother and I provide them with answers, they process what we've told them – then ask more questions. When my kids do that, it implies they don't believe our answer or there's more that we're not telling them. Just prior to age 12, I refrained from having conversations with DJ about his mother that reflected negatively on her. Each day closer to age 12 he began asking more and more direct questions – I answered them with the thought that he's still not able to fully understand all that he's asking. I certainly don't degrade her, but the answers don't always paint a flowery picture of his mom. However, my job as his dad is to raise him to be a man with character and discipline and at age 12, it sets a bad precedence for me to defend her actions when she's wrong. He senses I don't agree with all his mom does and doesn't do, but my position is known on disrespect. My character won't allow him to disrespect his mother, PERIOD! Most importantly, I think the key to R.E.R.R.L is to refrain from painting yourself as a hero-like figure that doesn't do anything wrong. Accepting responsibility for all that I have done, apologizing for it, then ensuring the situation is made right, is critical. At the end of the day, character and the way I treat others (including his mom) goes a long way with him. Moreover, the people I surround him with and the way that I love his sister and respect his grandparents helps him to see my character and ultimately builds his. **F|B**

CHAPTER 9 - FACTS & FINAL WORD

What happens if you can't get to an amicable agreement as co-parents? What happens if your children don't have their dad in their life? Hopefully, what I've shared has moved you, but if not, perhaps the illustration will.

Up front, I'll tell you that statistics are great so long as they don't come with an agenda or a slant. I've chosen not to include raw numbers from organizations in this book because the chart above and the concept that kids need their dad should sell itself. I could've taken each major factor in the chart and written many more chapters, but you've heard the real-life stories in this book that correlate with some of what you see above and maybe a couple of other things that you don't. Let's be honest – our children will fall into one or multiple categories by virtue of them being a human in today's society, even with a dad in the home. To this point, I needed some tough love from my dad as a teenager for making a couple of dumb decisions with significant consequences, but my dad's constant presence and life lessons ensured that I didn't stray far off of the beaten path. See Figure 1. 2017 Census Bureau.

THE FATHER ABSENCE CRISIS IN AMERICA

There is a crisis in America. According to the U.S. Census Bureau, 19.7 million children, more than 1 in 4, live without a father in the home. Consequently, there is a "father factor" in nearly all of the societal ills facing America today. Research shows when a child is raised in a father-absent home, he or she is affected in the following ways...

Source: 2017, U.S. Census Bureau. Data represent children living without a biological, step, or adoptive father.

POVERTY

 4X GREATER RISK OF **POVERTY**

TEEN PREGNANCY

7X MORE LIKELY TO BECOME **PREGNANT AS A TEEN**

BEHAVIORAL PROBLEMS

 MORE LIKELY TO HAVE **BEHAVIORAL PROBLEMS**

CHILD ABUSE

MORE LIKELY TO FACE **ABUSE AND NEGLECT**

MOM-CHILD HEALTH

 2X GREATER RISK OF **INFANT MORTALITY**

SUBSTANCE ABUSE

MORE LIKELY TO ABUSE **DRUGS AND ALCOHOL**

INCARCERATION

 MORE LIKELY TO GO **TO PRISON**

CHILD OBESITY

2X MORE LIKELY TO SUFFER **OBESITY**

CRIME

 MORE LIKELY TO COMMIT CRIME

EDUCATION

2X MORE LIKELY TO DROP OUT **OF HIGH SCHOOL**

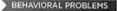

Statistics and charts aside, experience tells me that a factor leading to divorce has to do with one or both individuals being raised in a home that lacked a dad's projection of love, respect, and security for their mom. Children, teenagers, and young adults tend to emulate what they see, and if domestic abuse or crime is what they see, it's going to have an impact on them. Your son is less likely to degrade and abuse women if he wasn't raised seeing it. I can't stress enough to the dads and soon-to-be dads, you have every right to be there for your children - don't allow anything or anyone to keep you from them! Remember, your family name and reputation give your children a sense of identity, but your love and your presence help influence the people they will become. The world is a place our children can thrive in and yet, easily fall into traps. DO EVERYTHING YOU CAN TO HELP THEM AVOID THOSE TRAPS and ACHIEVE! LOVE is IMPORTANT! HISTORY is IMPORTANT! LITERACY is IMPORTANT! DIET & EXERCISE is IMPORTANT! LAND OWNERSHIP is IMPORTANT! FINANCIAL INDEPENDENCE is IMPORTANT! TRAVELING and CULTURE is IMPORTANT! It's your RESPONSIBILITY to lay the foundation and EQUIP them for the world – DO IT!

Moms, no disrespect intended but there are just some things you can't teach effectively-- KIDS NEED THEIR DADS from the time they're born through adulthood!!! Blocking your kids' blessings and upbringing by denying them access to a capable dad is repulsive. If you take your child to the hospital, their dad should know about it. If child is going on a date, he should know about it. Parent teacher conferences shouldn't be a secret, and discipline should be shared routinely as opposed to waiting until the child is in serious trouble and/or failing classes. When a teachable moment presents itself, he should be allowed to engage and help! Your child making the basketball team or cheerleading squad shouldn't be a surprise; they should be allowed to coach them and instill the courage to try. <u>At the end of the day, you have to love your children more than you hate the man that helped you conceive the child!</u>

When a person tears a ligament in their leg, it's safe to say, physical therapy is a requirement in order to facilitate the proper healing and use of the leg. Your children are no different!!! When you divorce or remove a parent from his/her life, the soul and emotions of the child are torn, and therapy is required to mend the soul. I'm not a doctor, therapist, or life coach, but I'd like to express to parents through my experience as a parent, there is absolutely nothing wrong with equipping your children with tools offered by a psychologist or counselor (like a "kid helper") to cope with turbulent times. All too often, couples will seek counseling and non-married couples will seek a friend to assist in figuring out ways to help keep a relationship going while the kids get nothing. This is criminal!! If professional help isn't affordable, seek non-profit organizations similar to the ones I've listed as resources on this project. If that's not possible, a life coach (pro-bono) or minister could also be a source of objective assistance.

If you recall, I grew up with two parents in the household, and my Dad's presence was felt even when he wasn't around. Therefore, it should be easy to see that when I started this journey as a single parent five years ago, I assumed there would be challenges raising my son without two parents in the home. In my marriage, I was always the disciplinarian and the one who was seen as the provider and protector. Being the sole parent in the home meant I was going to have to elevate and grow as a parent. It meant that teachable moments and discipline would be accompanied by compassion and sensitivity when the time called for it. It meant that I was going to have to learn how to be a dad to my daughter from a different state and giving love and discipline to her in a way that a nine year old can understand. There have been numerous obstacles in the way. My relationship isn't the best with the mother of my two children, but I've never given up on them. I've refused to go away and/or stop calling to speak to my daughter. Despite the fact that she lives in a different state, I haven't missed a birthday, and I routinely speak or meet with the administrators, teachers, and physician in my daughter's life. When I'm with my daughter, she's the center of my world.

I wish things were different, but my journey as a dad didn't start so great. Uncertainty about my then ex-wife's health and unborn son and myriad of other things I spoke of previously, all played a role. Thankfully, GOD blessed me with two healthy, beautiful children, a supportive circle of family and friends, and the mental capacity to learn from my mistakes. I see being a dad as a marathon rather than a 100-meter sprint. There's been enough drama in my first leg of the race between the mother of my children and I. Going forward, I'm hoping the greater good of our children moves to the fore-front, and we can begin raising them in a way that they see little to no space between us. In the next leg of the race, I look forward to the proms, science fairs, college orientations, and sporting events that come with the high school and college experience. Midway through the race is the period of time in which I get to watch my kids begin their journey as adults, as their careers, homeownership, and possibly grandchildren will be my new focus. Finally, the last leg of the race will consist of enjoying time with my grandkids while advising my kids on how to be better parents, invest wisely, and propel themselves to the next level their respective careers. I don't expect the road along the entire journey to be smooth, things in life rarely are – but helping my children through the many aspects of life is a responsibility I look forward to continuing until I'm no longer able. For all those who share those same sentiments, I applaud you, and hope to see you at the finish line. **F|B**

References

Blend: The Secret to Co-Parenting and Creating a Balanced Family; Mashonda Tifrere, Alicia Keys (Foreword by); 2018

Divorcing Dads: From Corruption to Connection; January 2018; website: http://www.thefatherhoodproject.org

The Fatherhood Initiative; January 2018; website: http://www.fatherhood.org

Fathers Resource and Networking Center (FRANC) – Champion for Children; January 2018; website: http://www.cfctb.org

He-Motions; T.D. Jakes; July 2013

A Father First: How My Life Became Bigger Than Basketball; Dwayne Wade; September 2012

Fatherhood: Rising to the Ultimate Challenge; Ethan Thomas, Nich Childs, and Tony Dungy; May 7, 2013

Divorce and Child Custody: Men Call Foul; This Is Life with Lisa Ling; November 2018; CNN website: http://www.cnn.com

US Census Bureau Father Statistics, 2017; http://www.census.gov